Andressa Vinha Zanuncio

DEFINITION OF THE NASAL ENDOSCOPIC REFERENCE POINT TO SURGICAL ACCESS

Andressa Vinha Zanuncio

DEFINITION OF THE NASAL ENDOSCOPIC REFERENCE POINT TO SURGICAL ACCESS

Anatomical Study

ScienciaScripts

Imprint

Cover image: www.ingimage.com

This book is a translation from the original published under ISBN 978-620-2-80874-3.

Publisher:
Sciencia Scripts
is a trademark of
International Book Market Service Ltd., member of OmniScriptum Publishing Group
17 Meldrum Street, Beau Bassin 71504, Mauritius
Printed at: see last page
ISBN: 978-620-3-40001-4

INDEX

To my parents, Teresa and
José, for their inspiration, pride and
unconditional support. To my husband,
Alexandre, for all the love.
To our daughter,
Cecília, for the example of
struggle and stamina and
for teaching me that we should never give up.

THANKS

To Professor Dr. Roberto Eustáquio dos Santos Guimarães, for his trust, incentive, friendship, and fundamental orientation in my medical formation and for the learning and scientific maturation. For his patience in understanding my personal difficulties.

To the Serviço de Verificação de Óbito da Universidade de São Paulo (SVOc-USP), which provided its laboratories for the research and received me as part of the team.

To the corpses, my deep respect and gratitude.

To the friends and employees of the Death Verification Service of the University of São Paulo (SVOc-USP) for all their help.

To the colleagues and employees of the Graduate Program in Sciences Applied to Surgery and Ophthalmology at the Medical School, UFMG.

To the Medical School of the Federal University of São João Del'Rey - CCO Campus, for understanding my absences.

To my husband Alexandre, for his support and incentive in the realization of my work, and to my daughter Cecília, my loves.

To my parents, Teresa and José, for all the love, dedication and example throughout my life. To Virgínia and Antônio, my dear siblings.

To everyone who has been on my side and, even without knowing it, has supported and encouraged me in some way.

1. INTRODUCTION

Diseases of the paranasal sinuses and skull base are often treated with operations aided by the use of the rigid nasal endoscope (nasal endoscopic operation). These operations have had great evolution with nasal endoscopy, new instruments and imaging exams. However, even with greater safety, there are a considerable number of complications of this technique, which can be serious, such as cerebrospinal fluid fistulas, pneumocephalus, intraorbital bleeding and partial or total loss of vision. In situations where there is distortion of the anatomy due to extensive nasal polyps, it is difficult to open and completely clean the sinuses.

The knowledge of the paranasal sinuses anatomy is primordial for the accomplishment of safe and efficient operations. The endoscopic operation, guided by computer, helps in the identification of anatomical structures, but it is an alternative of high price and little accessible in Brazil.

Endoscopic nasal surgery is used for the treatment of chronic rhinosinusitis, associated or not with nasal polyposis, resection of nasal and paranasal sinus tumors, malformations of the nasal cavity, such as choanal atresia, and various inflammatory and infectious diseases of the nasal cavity and paranasal sinuses. Access to the anterior skull base for the removal of tumors and treatment of neurological diseases is often performed through the nasal fossa. Technological advances in surgical instruments, diagnostic imaging methods, and fiber optics allow this type of operation to be performed more safely and effectively.

The operation guided by nasal endoscope (endoscopic nasal operation) is performed with 0°, 30°, 45° or 70° optics for visualization of the nasal cavity and paranasal sinuses according to the sinus affected, which allows access to the maxillary, ethmoid, frontal and sphenoid sinuses and the anterior cranial base. Noble structures such as the optic nerve, carotid artery and ocular globes can be iatrogenically injured by their proximity to the surgical site and anatomical variations of these sinuses can favor inadvertent injury. The fragility of the ethmoid sinus roof at the base of the skull can lead to pneumocephalus and cerebrospinal fluid fistulas. Imaging examinations with a detailed study of the sinus anatomy before the surgical procedure, consultation of these examinations during the operation, and training of the surgeon minimize these risks. The sinus anatomy can be used for personal identification, analogous to a fingerprint, due to its individual variation.

Morbidity can be reduced with detailed knowledge of paranasal sinus anatomy. In addition, the greatest surgical success and cure of disease can be achieved when all paranasal sinuses are adequately approached, especially the posterior ethmoid and sphenoid sinuses, where the greatest complications occur.

The knowledge of fixed measurements, which vary little in relation to characteristics such as gender, ethnicity, age, weight, and height, such as the distance from the posterior wall of the maxillary sinus to the anterior cranial base, for example, would give surgeons more security when approaching the posterior sinuses, minimizing iatrogenesis. These measures have not been described in the literature.

The hypothesis of a fixed distance between the posterior wall of the maxillary sinus and the skull base has been shown by observations in surgical practice to facilitate nasal endoscopic operations.

2. OBJECTIVES

The purpose of this study was to measure the distances from the posterior wall of the right and left maxillary sinuses to the anterior cranial base and compare them with the socio-demographic characteristics of interest; to define other reference points for endoscopic surgical access; to compare the anatomical variations of the measured reference points in relation to gender, height, weight, age, and ethnicity in cadavers; and to detail a new anatomical reference point to perform more safely operations of the paranasal sinuses and the anterior cranial base.

3. LITERATURE REVIEW

The literature review was carried out in the main otorhinolaryngology journals and related areas through pubmed. Scientific papers reporting measurements of the paranasal sinuses or measurements of the anterior cranial base are scarce, but the medical literature presents studies in cadavers with evaluation of the characteristics of the paranasal sinuses, evaluation of the operative technique of functional endoscopic sinus surgery (FESS) and its complications. Knowledge of the anatomy of the paranasal sinuses allows a better approach to them during endoscopic nasal surgery. CT scans allow a previous study of the anatomical characteristics of that individual, taking into account the individual variations of this anatomy. A study reviewing 512 CT scans of the sinuses (1024 sides) showed diverse variations emphasizing the importance of knowledge of individual variations in preventing complications (KANTARCI, M. 2004).Endoscopic nasal operation is an added surgical option as a form of treatment for various disorders of the paranasal sinuses and nasal cavity, such as in chronic rhinosinusitis, nasal polyposis, skull base diseases, septal deviations, with lower morbidity and greater safety (LUONG and MARPLE 2006).A study of 48 cadaver heads evaluating 96 sphenoid sinuses in an Asian population defined characteristics of these sinuses, the most common type being the selar. Forty-five percent (45%) individuals had a dominant sphenoid sinus and the Asian population showed a higher incidence of posterior ethmoid cells, situated cephalad to the sphenoid sinuses, offering a higher risk of optic nerve injury in this population. However, the measurements of the sphenoid sinuses or their relationship to the anterior wall of the skull have not been cited (TAN, 2007).Anatomical variations of the posterior ethmoid and sphenoid sinuses in 50 CT scans of the facial sinuses showed aspects of anatomical variations, such as the presence of Onodi's cell, variations of the sphenoid sinuses, and dehiscence of the sphenoid wall in the topography of the optic nerve, among others, emphasizing the great variation in the anatomy of the paranasal sinuses (SCUTARI and BÂLDEA 2010).Patients with chronic rhinosinusitis and nasal polyposis present important symptoms of nasal obstruction (TAN and LANE 2009) interfering directly in their quality of life and causing recurrent acute infections, increasing the morbidity of these patients. There is an improvement in the quality of life of patients with chronic rhinosinusitis, associated or not with polyposis, and improvement of asthma symptoms in patients undergoing FESS (BUNZEN and CAMPOS 2006).The fundamental principles of endoscopic nasal operation and knowledge of anatomy allow a greater success of FESS (STAMM 2002) and a smaller number of complications.Computer guided operation was idealized to assist the surgeon in the precise location of anatomical structures during surgery, providing more safety for the patient and the doctor. The operations that had the greatest need for the system were those performed to access lesions at the skull base, in revisionary polyps with altered anatomy and in the region of the frontal recess (STAMM, PIGNATARI, SEBUSIANI and GALATI 2002 and HEMMERDINGER,

JACOBS, 2005).

All are situations where noble structures are close or the anatomical references are distorted. In Brazil, the use of computer-guided surgery is still an inaccessible and high-cost resource, making the use of this tool unfeasible in clinical practice.Nasal endoscopic operations allow a safe access and with lessormorbidity for skull base lesions and sinus disorders (LUBBE and SEMPLE 2008). A group of 15 patients undergoing endonasal operation for resection of pituitary tumor was compared to another group of 15 patients undergoing conventional operation. The group undergoing endoscopic surgery had shorter hospital stay, less pain, less bleeding and shorter recovery time (CASLER and DOOLITTLE 2005). The endonasal technique for addressing skull base lesions is an increasingly used technique, recurrence of nasal polyps, narrowing of the frontal recess and failure of maxillary antrostomy are causes of operative reintervention in FESS (MUSY and KOUNTAKIS 2004). Postoperative complications and disease recurrence generate an average of 18% reinterventions in postoperative FESS (TAN and CHANDRA 2010).

Measurements in 151 CT scans of the ethmoid fovea of the paranasal sinuses were taken and compared for right and left sides. Inadvertent lesions of this region can cause cranial compromise. Five different shapes were found, showing the anatomical variation of the ethmoid fovea (JONES, ALMAHDI and BHALLA 2001). Therefore, a fixed anatomical measurement would help the ESF with more safety and fewer complications.

4. MATERIAL AND METHODS

4.1. Description of the study

The study was approved by the Research Ethics Committee of UFMG (Federal University of Minas Gerais) under opinion number 0591.0.203.000-8 (Appendix 2).

The study was conducted to determine anatomical reference points for access to the anterior cranial base, by measuring the distance from the posterior wall of the maxillary sinus to the anterior cranial base, based on operative observations, where distances greater than 2cm were found.

The corpses were autopsied at the Serviço de Verificação de Óbitos da Universidade de São Paulo (SVOc-USP), in July 2010, because there were no Serviços de Verificação de Óbitos in the state of Minas Gerais, making it impossible to carry out the study. The cadavers were registered in a form containing age, ethnicity, gender and height (Appendix 1). Regarding ethnicity, the corpses were divided into two groups, whites and browns; the blacks were included in the brown group, as this is the standard classification of the SVOc-USP. The identification of the bodies and the information concerning them were kept confidential. The distances in the nasal cavities were measured, all performed by the researcher, the author of this study. We opened the medial wall of the maxillary sinus, dissected the anterior and posterior ethmoid sinuses and the sphenoid sinus (Figures 1 to 6), to identify the point where the deflection of the skull base begins to form the anterior wall of the sphenoid, where there is often an angle close to 90 degrees (point called 90° angle - Δ 90°) and measured from this point to three points on the posterior wall of the maxillary sinus. The dissection was performed with microsurgical material by nasal endoscopy with 0° optics, and recorded on DVD in an attached camera. The structure for the study was assembled in the necropsy room of the SVOc-USP, using a video camera, notebook, aspirator, light source, surgical instruments, zero degree optics and light cable. The cadavers, after the necropsy to verify death, were taken on stretchers to this region of the room and the paranasal sinuses were dissected, with subsequent measurements being taken.

Measurements and changes of major significance were photographed, videotaped, and kept in the researcher's file. The forceps used for dissection are delicate micro forceps used in nasal endoscopic operations. No biological material was removed from the cadavers.

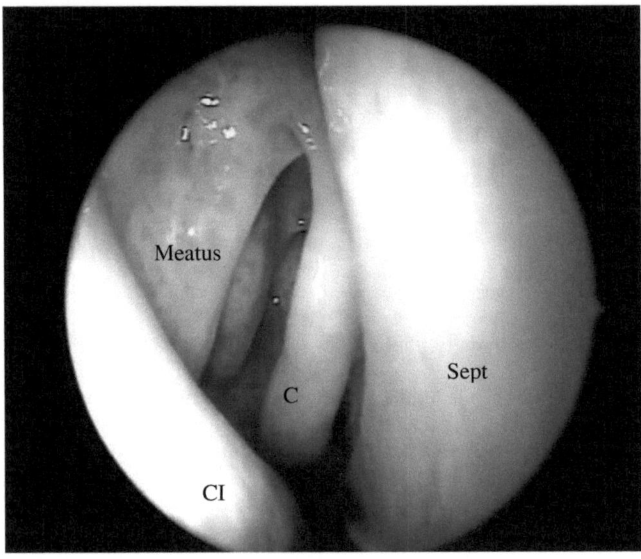

FIGURE 1: Right nasal cavity (CM: middle turbinate / CI: lower turbinate)

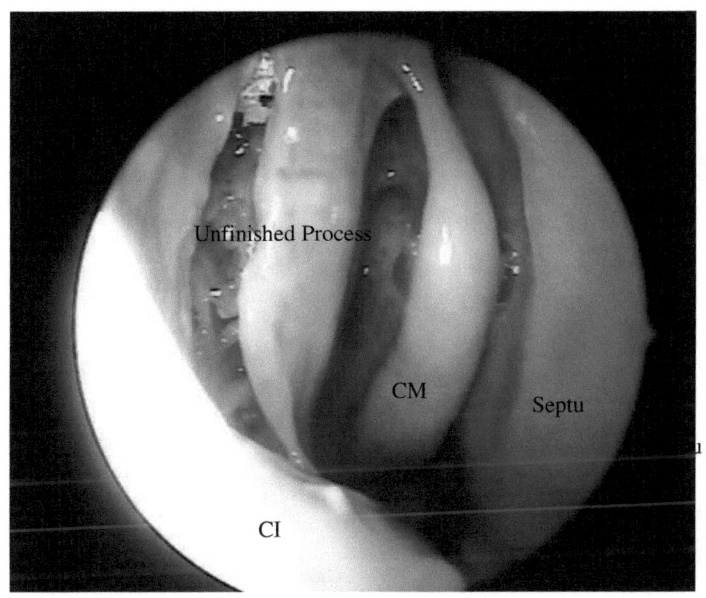

FIGURE 2: Beginning of dissection (CM: middle turbinate / CI: inferior turbinate)

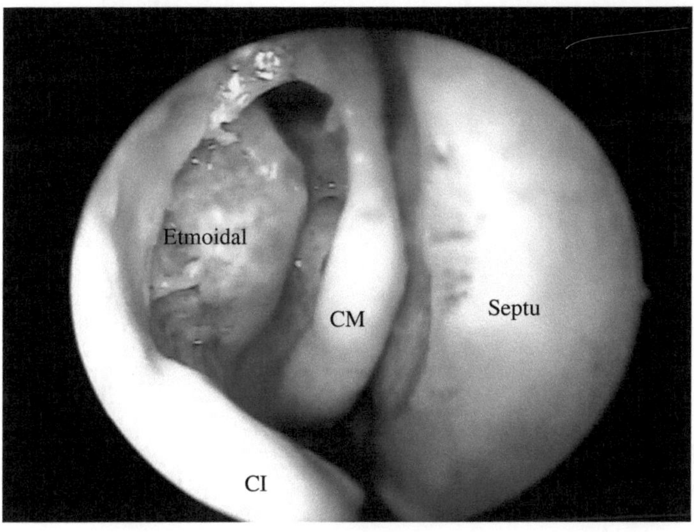

FIGURE 3: Ethmoidal bulla (CM: middle turbinate / CI: lower turbinate)

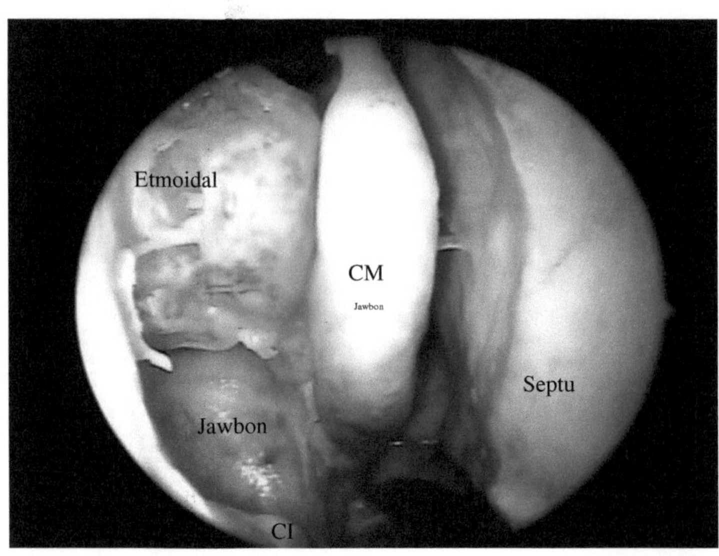

FIGURE 4: Maxillary sinus exposure (CM: middle turbinate / CI: lower turbinate)

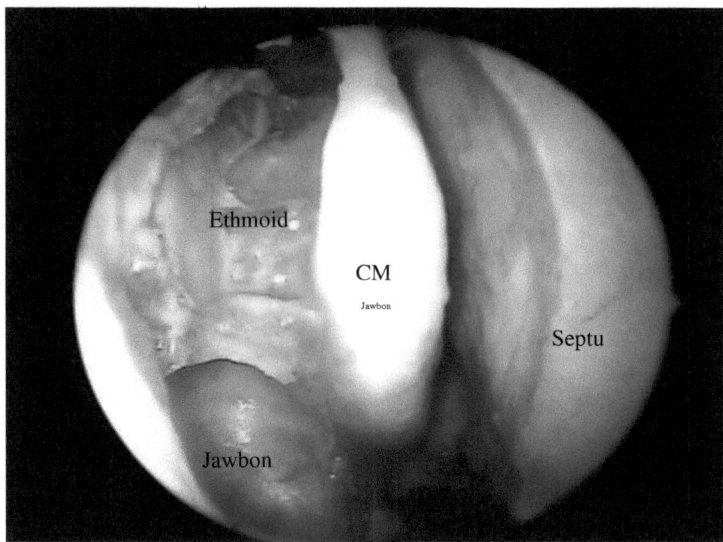

FIGURE 5: Exposure of the ethmoid sinus (CM: middle turbinate)

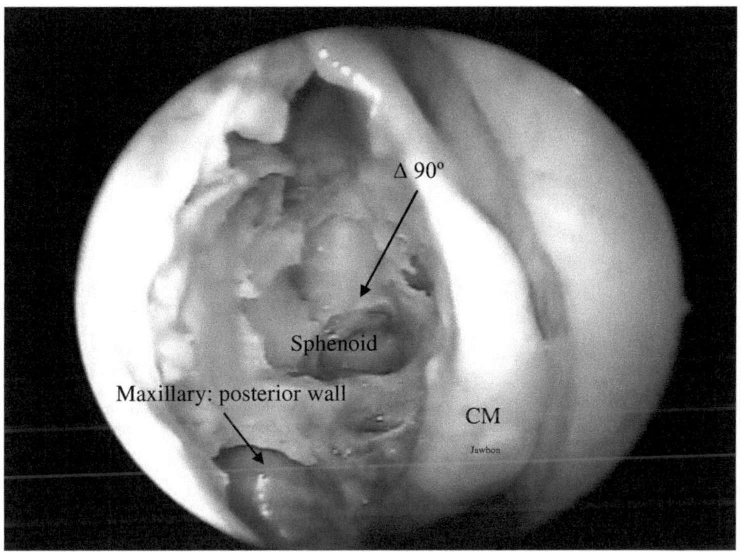

FIGURE 6: Exposure of the sphenoid sinus. The arrow points to the 90° angle.

The material studied are the values of the measurements performed in cadavers, from which the paranasal sinuses were dissected (Figure 7). The measurements are: superior, middle and inferior points of the posterior wall of the maxillary sinus up to the 90º angle; superior, middle and inferior points of the posterior wall of the maxillary sinus up to the nasal spine; frontal sinus recess up to the nasal spine; frontal sinus recess up to the 90º angle; 90º angle up to the anterior nasal spine, based on a previously stipulated protocol. The nine measurements under study were evaluated on the right and left sides and only the measurements from the Δ 90° to the upper, middle and lower points of the posterior maxillary sinus wall were evaluated in both quantitative and categorical form. The variables, the form, and the observations on these variables are presented in Table 1.We chose to exclude measurements 1, 2, 3, 4, 5, and 7 and perform the work based on measurements 6, 8, and 9, since the first six suffered variation in relation to socio-demographic characteristics, and the three selected did not suffer variation in relation to socio-demographic characteristics and had greater relevance.

The three selected measures were dichotomized into two groups: greater than or equal to two and less than two, because in the operative practice it was observed that the distances were in general greater than or equal to two.

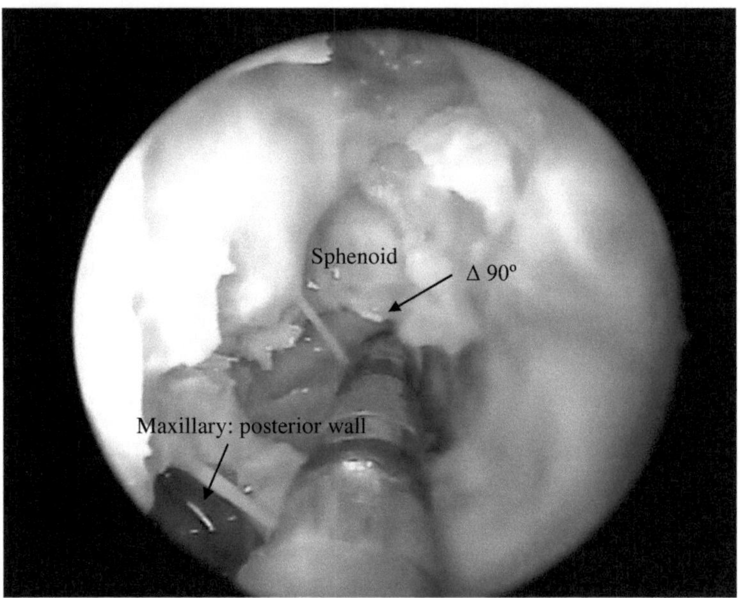

FIGURE 7: Carrying out the measurements on the cadavers.

TABLE 1. Name and form of the response variables

Name of Response Variables	Form	Note
1- Δ 90º to anterior nasal spine	Quantitativ e	-
2- Frontal recess to the anterior nasal spine	Quantitativ e	-
3- Posterior maxillary wall up to the anterior nasal spine	Quantitativ e	-
4- Posterior maxillary middle wall to the anterior nasal spine	Quantitativ e	-
5- Posterior maxillary wall inferior to the anterior nasal spine	Quantitativ e	-
6- Δ 90º to the maxillary posterior superior wall	Quantitativ e/ categorical	Dichotomized at ≥ 2 or < 2
7- Δ 90º to the front recess	Quantitativ e	-
8- Δ 90º to the posterior medial maxillary wall	Quantitativ e/ categorical	Dichotomized at ≥ 2 or < 2
9- Δ 90º to the lower posterior maxillary wall	Quantitativ e/ categorical	Dichotomized at ≥ 2 or < 2

How the covariates were evaluated in relation to the three response variables are shown in Table 2.

TABLE 2. Covariates and form under study.

Covariates	Form	Note
Gender (Male and Female)	Categorical	-
Height (meters)	Quantitative	-
Age (years)	Quantitative	-
Ethnicity (white and brown)	Categorical	-
Weight (Kg)	Quantitative	-

The inclusion of the cadaver in the study was recorded in the necropsy report, as well as information about the procedure for research purposes. We studied 60 randomly selected cadavers of different ages, ethnicities, statures and of both genders, aged over 17 years. Corpses with suspected death from external injuries were excluded and sent by the SVOc-USP to the Medico-Legal Institute.

4.2. Statistical Analysis

The descriptive results were obtained using frequencies and percentages for the characteristics of the various categorical variables and obtaining measures of central tendency (mean and median) and measures of dispersion (standard deviation) for quantitative variables. In this type of chart, the circles indicate cadavers considered to have extreme values (outliers), that is, very different from the values presented by the other cadavers. The beginning of the box represents the first quartile, i.e., that 25% of the observations are below this value. The center line represents the median, indicating that 50% of the values are above and 50% are below this value. The end of the box represents the third quartile, indicating that 75% of the observations are below this value (TRIOLA, 2005).

4.3. Comparisons with measurements made

Pearson's correlation coefficient (r) was used to compare the quantitative measures with the quantitative characteristics (age, height, weight, and Body Mass Index - BMI).Student's t-tests were used for comparisons of the quantitative measurements with gender and ethnicity, since the usual assumptions of this test were met (normality - Shapiro-Wilk and homoscedasticity - Levene) (TRIOLA, 2005).Comparisons of the measurement of the 90° angle (Δ 90°) to the posterior wall of the jaw categorized with gender and ethnicity were performed by contingency tables and Fisher's test was applied. The analyses were performed in the R *software*, public domain, at 5% significance level.

5. RESULTS

5.1. Descriptive Analysis

A higher frequency of males (55%) and whites (78.3%) was observed in the 60 cadavers (Table 1).

TABLE 1: Gender and ethnicity description

Features	**Frequency**	
	n	**%**
Genre		
Male	33	*55,0*
Female	27	*45,0*
Ethnicity		
White	47	*78,3*
Brown	13	*21,7*

The cadavers were, on average, 64 years old, 1.70 meters, 67.1 kilos, and a BMI of 22.5 (Table 2). Regarding age, the standard deviation is 18.2, with a minimum of 17 years and a maximum of 97 years, and 25% were approximately less than 54 years old (1st quartile), 50% were less than 65 years old (median), and 75% were at least 78 years old (3rd quartile).

TABLE 2: Description of the cadavers regarding age, height and weight

Feature	n	Average	D.P.	Minimum	1ST Q	Median	3RD Q	Maximum
Age (years)	60	64,2	18,2	17,0	53,5	64,5	78,0	97,0
Height (meters)	60	1,7	0,1	1,6	1,7	1,7	1,8	1,9
Weight (kg)	60	67,1	10,1	40,0	60,0	68,0	74,5	88,0
BMI	60	22,5	2,9	15,6	20,1	23,1	24,7	27,3

n: number of observations, S.D.: standard deviation, 1Q: 1st quartile, 3Q: 3rd quartile.

The cadavers were between 48 and 88 years old, between 1.70 and 1.75 meters tall, weighed between 60 and 80 kilos, and had a BMI between 18 and 26 (Figures 8, 10, 12 and 14).

The *box-plots of* age, height, weight, and BMI are shown in Figures 9, 11, 13 e 15.

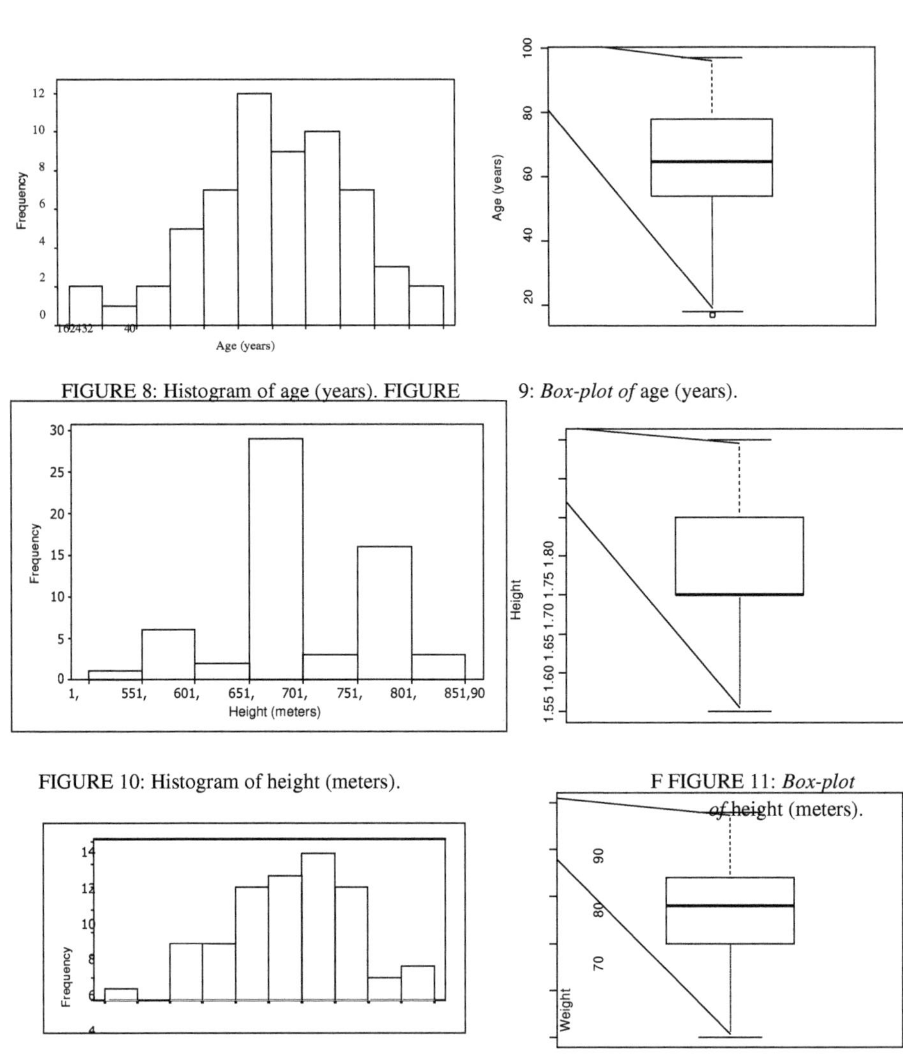

FIGURE 8: Histogram of age (years). FIGURE 9: *Box-plot of* age (years).

FIGURE 10: Histogram of height (meters).

F FIGURE 11: *Box-plot of* height (meters).

FIGURE 12: Histogram of weight (kilograms). FIGURE 13: *Box-plot of* weight (kilograms).

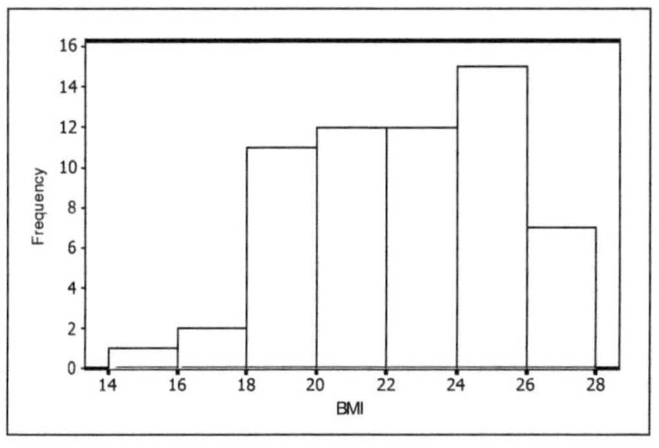

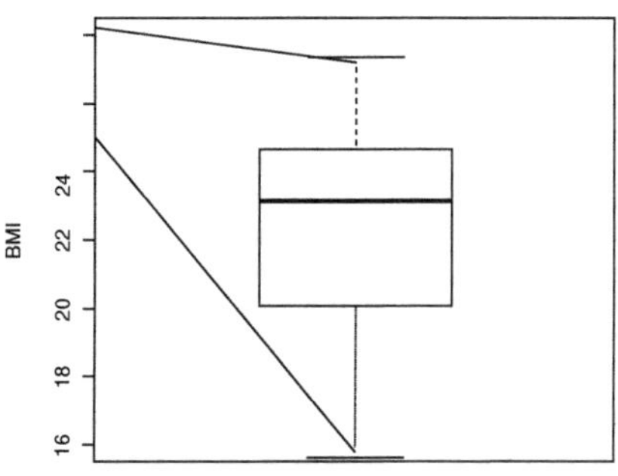

FIGURE 14: Histogram of the BMI. FIGURE 15: *Box-plot* of BMI.

The descriptive statistics of the three response variables evaluated on the right and left sides are presented in Table 3. On the right side, the cadavers had on average, 2.1cm from Δ 90° to the upper posterior maxillary wall; 1.9cm from Δ 90° to the middle posterior maxillary wall, and 1.7cm from Δ 90° to the lower posterior maxillary wall. On the left side, the cadavers had 2.2 cm, 1.7cm, and 1.6 cm, respectively.

TABLE 3: Description of the descriptive statistics on the right and left sides

Features	**n**	**Avera ge**	**D.P.**	**Min.**	**1Q**	**Med.**	**3Q**	**Max.**
Law								
Δ 90° to upper back wall*	60	2,1	0,3	1,5	2,0	2,0	2,5	3,0
Δ 90° to posterior medial wall*	60	1,9	0,5	1,0	1,5	2,0	2,0	3,0
Δ 90° to lower back wall*	60	1,7	0,5	0,5	1,5	1,5	2,0	2,5
Left								
Δ 90° to upper back wall*	60	2,2	0,4	1,5	2,0	2,0	2,5	3,0
Δ 90° to posterior medial wall*	60	1,7	0,4	1,0	1,5	2,0	2,0	2,5
Δ 90° to lower back wall*	60	1,6	0,4	0,5	1,5	1,5	2,0	2,5

n: number of observations, S.D.: standard deviation, min: minimum, 1Q: 1st Quartile, med: median, 3Q: 3rd Quartile, max: maximum. Refers to the maxillary sinus.

Box-plots illustrating the quartiles, variability and the presence of *outliers* for each of the three response variables per side are presented in Figures 16 through 18.

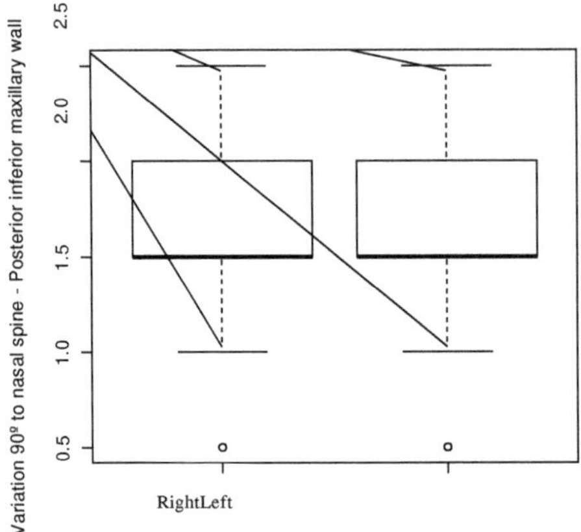

FIGURE 18: Variation of Δ 90° to the lower posterior maxillary wall

Regarding the categorized measurements, 91.7% of the cadavers had the measurement of the Δ 90º to the upper posterior maxillary wall greater than or equal to 2. Sixty-one point seven (61.7%) and 51.7% of the cadavers had on the right and left side, respectively, the distance from the Δ 90° to the middle posterior maxillary wall greater than or equal to 2. Forty-six point seven (46.7%) and 41.7% of the cadavers had on the right and left side, respectively, the distance from the Δ 90° to the lower posterior wall of the jaw greater than or equal to 2 (Table 4).

TABLE 4: Categorized description of the measurements from Δ 90° to the upper posterior, middle and lower jaw wall

Features	Frequency			
	Right side		Left Side	
	n	**%**	**n**	**%**
Δ 90° to posterior medial maxillary wall				
< 2	23	*38,3*	29	*48,3*
≥ 2	37	*61,7*	31	*51,7*
Δ 90° to lower posterior maxillary wall				
< 2	32	*53,3*	35	*58,3*
≥ 2	28	*46,7*	25	*41,7*
Δ 90° to upper posterior maxillary wall				
< 2	5	*8,3*	5	*8,3*
≥ 2	55	*91,7*	55	*91,7*

5.2. Side-by-side comparisons

There was a difference with statistical significance between the sides only in the measurement of the Δ 90° to the middle posterior maxillary wall. The difference between the means of this characteristic between the sides is only 0.2 cm (1.9-1.7 cm), with the left side being smaller than the right (Table 5).

TABLE 5: Comparison of the right and left side response variables

Features	**Sides**						
	Right			**Left**			**p**
	Average	**D.P.**	**Med.**	**Average**	**D.P.**	**Med.**	
Δ 90° to upper back wall*	2,1	0,3	2,0	2,2	0,4		2, 00,277 1
Δ 90° to posterior medial wall*	1,9	0,5	2,0	1,7	0,4	2,0	**0,0201**
Δ 90° to lower back wall*	1,7	0,5	1,5	1,6	0,4		1, 50,417 2

S.D.: Standard deviation, Med: Median, 1: Paired t-test. Referring to the maxillary sinus.

5.3. Comparisons of the characteristics with the response variables by right and left side.

5.3.1. 90° angle (Δ 90°) to the upper posterior jaw wall

a) Right Side - Quantitative

No associations were observed between age, height, weight, and BMI ($p>0.05$) (Table 6) or gender and ethnicity of the cadavers ($p > 0.05$) (Table 7) with the measurement of the Δ 90° to the upper posterior maxillary wall.

TABLE 6: Correlation between Δ 90° to the upper posterior maxillary wall on the right side with age, height, weight, and BMI

Features	**r**	**Value-p**
Age (years)	0,031	0,8141
Height (meters)	0,054	0,6811
Weight (kg)	-0,162	0,2171
BMI	-0,227	0,0811

1: Pearson's correlation coefficient.

TABLE 7: Comparison of Δ 90° to the upper posterior maxillary wall on the right side with gender and ethnicity

Features	**n**	**Average**	**D.P.**	**Min.**	**1Q**	**Median**	**3Q**	**Max.**	**Value-p**
Genre									
Male	33	2,1	0,3	1,5	2,0	2,0	2,5	2,5	0,4821
Female	27	2,1	0,3	1,5	2,0	2,0	2,5	3,0	
Ethnicity									
White	47	2,1	0,3	1,5	2,0	2,0	2,5	2,5	0,9871
Brown	13	2,1	0,4	1,5	2,0	2,0	2,5	3,0	

n: number of observations, S.D.: standard deviation, 1Q: 1st quartile, 3Q: 3rd quartile,
1: Student's t-test.

b) Right Side - Categorical

Regarding the comparisons of the categorized measurement from Δ 90° to the posterior superior wall of the maxilla on the right side in relation to age, height, weight, and BMI, no association was observed ($p > 0.05$) (Table 8).

TABLE 8: Comparison of the categorized measurements from Δ 90° to the posterior maxillary superior wall on the right side with age, height, weight, and BMI

Features	**Δ 90° to upper posterior maxillary wall**						**p-value**
	≤ 2			**>2**			
	Mean	**P.D.**	**Median**		**P.D.**	**Median**	
Age (years)	63,0	17,9	74,0	64,4	18,4	64,0	0,8671
Height (meters)	1,7	0,1	1,7	1,7	0,1	1,7	0,6471
Weight (kg)	70,6	6,9	68,0	66,8	10,3	68,0	0,4271
BMI	23,4	2,6	23,5	22,5	2,9	23,1	0,5061

S.D.: standard deviation; 1: Student's t-test.

Comparisons of the measurement of Δ 90° to the upper posterior maxillary wall categorized on the right side in relation to gender and race of the cadavers are presented in Table 9. No association is observed between these characteristics and the measurement of Δ 90° to the upper posterior maxillary wall categorized on the right side ($p > 0.05$).

TABLE 9: Comparison of the categorized measurements from Δ 90° to the upper posterior maxillary wall on the right side with gender and ethnicity

Features	Δ 90° to upper back wall jaw				Value-p	OR	95% CI
	≤ 2		>2				
	n	%	n	%			
Genre							
Male	3	9,1	30	90,9	1,0001	1,3	0,2 a 11,8
Female	2	7,4	25	92,6		1,0	
Ethnicity							
White	4	8,5	43	91,5	1,0001	1,1	0,1 a 28,8
Brown	1	7,7	12	92,3		1,0	

1: Fisher's test.

c) Left Side - Quantitative

No associations were observed between age, height, weight, and BMI ($p>0.05$) (Table 10) or gender and ethnicity of the cadavers ($p > 0.05$) (Table 11) with the measurement of the Δ 90° to the upper posterior maxillary wall.

TABLE 10: Correlation between Δ 90° to the upper posterior maxillary wall on the left side with age, height, weight, and BMI

Features	r	Value-p
Age (years)	0,040	0,7621
Height (meters)	0,159	0,2251
Weight (kg)	-0,004	0,9761
BMI	-0,107	0,4151

1: Pearson's correlation coefficient.

TABLE 11: Comparison of Δ 90° to the upper posterior maxillary wall on the left side with gender and ethnicity

Feature	n	Average	D.P.	Min.	1Q	Median	3Q	Max.	Value-p
Genre									
Male	33	2,1	0,4	1,5	2,0	2,0	2,5	3,0	1,000 1
Female	27	2,1	0,3	1,5	2,0	2,0	2,5	3,0	
Ethnicity									
White	47	2,2	0,4	1,5	2,0	2,0	2,5	3,0	0,304 1
Brown	13	2,1	0,3	1,5	2,0	2,0	2,0	3,0	

n: number of observations, S.D.: standard deviation, 1Q: 1st quartile, 3Q: 3rd quartile, 1: Student's t-test.

d) Left Side - Categorical

There was no association between the categorized measurements from Δ 90° to the posterior superior maxillary wall on the left side in relation to age, height, weight, and BMI ($p > 0.05$) (Table 12) and in relation to gender and ethnicity ($p > 0.05$) (Table 13).

TABLE 12: Comparison of the categorized measurements from Δ 90° to the upper posterior maxillary wall on the left side with age, height, weight, and BMI

Feature	Δ 90° to upper posterior maxillary wall						Value-p
	≤2			>2			
	Average	D.P.	Median	Average	D.P.	Median	
Age (years)	67,8	13,8	73,0	63,9	18,7	63,0	0,6521
Height (meters)	1,7	0,1	1,7	1,7	0,1	1,7	0,1671
Weight (kg)	63,4	7,9	65,0	67,5	10,3	69,0	0,3931
BMI	22,4	1,8	22,5	22,5	3,0	23,1	0,9091

S.D.: standard deviation; 1: Student's t-test.

TABLE 13: Comparison of the categorized measurements from Δ 90° to the upper posterior maxillary wall on the left side with gender and ethnicity

Features	Δ 90° to the upper posterior maxillary wall				Value-p	OR	95% CI
	≤ 2		>2				
	n	%	n	%			
Genre							
Male	3	9,1	30	90,9	1,0001	1,3	0,2 a 11,8
Female	2	7,4	25	92,6		1,0	
Ethnicity							
White	4	8,5	43	91,5	1,0001	1,1	0,1 a 28,8
Brown	1	7,7	12	92,3		1,0	

1: Fisher's test.

Ten (10%) of the 60 cadavers had the measurement from Δ 90° to the posterior superior maxillary wall less than 2cm and more than 1.5cm.

5.3.2. Δ 90° to the posterior medial maxillary wall

5.3.2.1. Quantitative right side

No associations of the Δ 90° to the middle posterior maxillary wall measurement were observed with age, height, weight, and BMI ($p > 0.05$) (Table 14) and with gender and ethnicity ($p > 0.05$) (Table 15).

TABLE 14: Correlation of the measurement of Δ 90° to the medial posterior maxillary wall on the right side with age, height, weight and BMI

Features	r	Value-p
Age (years)	-0,145	0,2681
Height (meters)	0,061	0,6431
Weight (kg)	0,043	0,7461

BMI	0,014	0,9161

1: Pearson's correlation coefficient.

TABLE 15: Comparison of the measurement of Δ 90° to the medial posterior maxillary wall on the right side with gender and ethnicity

Features	n	Average	D.P.	Min.	1Q	Median	3Q	Max.	Value-p
Genre									
Male	33	1,9	0,5	1,0	1,5	2,0	2,3	3,0	0,5851
Female	27	1,9	0,6	1,0	1,5	2,0	2,0	3,0	
Ethnicity									
White	47	1,9	0,5	1,0	1,5	2,0	2,0	3,0	0,8021
Brown	13	1,9	0,5	1,0	1,5	2,0	2,3	3,0	

n: number of observations, S.D.: standard deviation, 1Q: 1st quartile, 3Q: 3rd quartile,
1: Student's t-test.

5.3.2.2. Right side - categorical

No association of the categorized measurement from Δ 90° to the medial posterior maxillary wall on the right side was observed in relation to age, height, weight, and BMI ($p > 0.05$) (Table 16) and in relation to gender and ethnicity ($p > 0.05$) (Table 17).

TABLE 16: Comparison of the categorized measurements from Δ 90° to the medial posterior maxillary wall on the right side with age, height, weight, and BMI

Features	Δ 90° to the posterior medial wall of the jaw						Value-p
	< 2			≥ 2			
	Average	D.P.	Median	Average	D.P.	Median	
Age (years)	63,4	22,2	67,0	64,7	15,6	63,0	0,7921
Height (meters)	1,7	0,1	1,7	1,7	0,1	1,7	0,4341
Weight (kg)	68,4	10,6	68,0	66,3	9,9	70,0	0,4361
BMI	22,7	2,7	23,2	22,4	3,0	22,5	0,7601

S.D.: standard deviation; 1: Student's t-test.

TABLE 17: Comparison of the categorized measurements from Δ 90° to the medial posterior maxillary wall on the right side with gender and ethnicity

Features	Δ 90° to the posterior medial wall of the jaw				Value-p	OR	95% CI
	< 2		≥ 2				
	n	%	n	%			
Genre							
Male	12	36,4	21	63,6	0,9362	0,8	0,3 a 2,7
Female	11	40,7	16	59,3		1,0	
Ethnicity							
White	18	38,3	29	61,7	1,0001	1,0	0,2 a 4,2
Brown	5	38,5	8	61,5		1,0	

1: Fisher's test; 2: Chi-square test with Yates' correction.

5.3.2.3. Quantitative left side

No associations were observed between age, height, weight, and BMI (p>0.05) (Table 18) or gender and ethnicity of the cadavers (p > 0.05) (Table 19) with the measurement of the Δ 90° to the middle posterior maxillary wall.

TABLE 18: Correlation between the measurement of Δ 90° to the middle posterior maxillary wall on the left side with age, height, weight and BMI

Features	r	Value-p
Age (years)	-0,093	0,4801
Height (meters)	0,125	0,3421
Weight (kg)	0,170	0,1941
BMI	0,123	0,3471

1: Pearson's correlation coefficient.

TABLE 19: Comparison of the measurement of Δ 90° to the medial posterior maxillary wall on the left side with gender and ethnicity

Features	n	Average	D.P.	Min.	1Q	Median	3Q	Max.	Value-p
Genre									
Male	33	1,8	0,4	1,0	1,5	2,0	2,0	2,5	0,5171
Female	27	1,7	0,4	1,0	1,5	1,5	2,0	2,5	
Ethnicity									
White	47	1,7	0,4	1,0	1,5	2,0	2,0	2,5	0,5011
Brown	13	1,7	0,5	1,0	1,3	1,5	2,0	2,5	

n: number of observations, S.D.: standard deviation, 1Q: 1st quartile, 3Q: 3rd quartile, 1: Student's t-test.

5.3.2.4. Left side - categorical

There was no association between the categorized measurements from Δ 90° to the medial posterior maxillary wall on the left side in relation to age, height, weight, and BMI ($p > 0.05$) (Table 20) and in relation to gender and ethnicity ($p > 0.05$) (Table 21).

TABLE 20: Comparison of the categorized measurements from Δ 90° to the maxillary medial posterior wall on the left side with age, height, weight, and BMI

Features	Δ 90° to the posterior medial wall of the jaw						Value-p
	< 2			≥ 2			
	Average	D.P.	Median	Average	D.P.	Median	
Age (years)	67,9	15,5	70,0	60,8	20,1	62,0	0,1301
Height (meters)	1,7	0,1	1,7	1,7	0,1	1,7	0,2031
Weight (kg)	65,8	9,0	67,0	68,4	11,0	70,0	0,3121
BMI	22,4	2,5	21,1	22,6	3,3	24,1	0,7451

S.D.: standard deviation; 1: Student's t-test

TABLE 21: Comparison of the categorized measurements from Δ 90° to the maxillary posterior medial wall on the left side with gender and ethnicity

Features	**Δ 90° to the back wall maxillary average**				**Value-p**	**OR**	**95% CI**
	< 2		**≥ 2**				
	n	**%**	**n**	**%**			
Genre							
Male	14	42,4	19	57,6	0,4512	0,6	0,2 a 1,9
Female	15	55,6	12	44,4		1,0	
Ethnicity							
White	21	44,7	26	55,3	0,4552	0,5	0,2 a 2,1
Brown	8	61,5	5	38,5		1,0	

2: Chi-square test with Yates' correction.

5.3.3. Δ 90° to the lower posterior maxillary wall

5.3.3.1. Right side - quantitative

No associations of the Δ 90° to the lower posterior maxillary wall measurement were observed with age, height, weight, and BMI ($p > 0.05$) (Table 22) and with gender and ethnicity ($p > 0.05$) (Table 23).

TABLE 22: Correlation between the measurement of Δ 90° to the lower posterior maxillary wall on the right side with age, height, weight and BMI

Features	**r**	**Value-p**
Age (years)	-0,237	0,0681
Height (meters)	0,138	0,2951
Weight (kg)	-0,005	0,9671
BMI	-0,088	0,5021

1: Pearson's correlation coefficient.

TABLE 23: Comparison of the measurement of Δ 90° to the lower posterior maxillary wall on the right side with gender and ethnicity

Features	n	Avera ge	D.P	Min.	1Q	Median	3Q	Max.	Value-p
Genre									
Male	33	1,8	0,5	1,0	1,5	2,0	2,0	2,5	0,3171
Female	27	1,6	0,5	0,5	1,5	1,5	2,0	2,5	
Ethnicity									
White	47	1,7	0,5	0,5	1,5	1,5	2,0	2,5	0,8001
Brown	13	1,7	0,5	1,0	1,3	2,0	2,0	2,5	

n: number of observations, S.D.: standard deviation, 1Q: 1st quartile, 3Q: 3rd quartile, 1: Student's t-test.

5.3.3.2 Right side - categorical

There was no association between the categorized measurements from Δ 90° to the posterior inferior wall of the right-sided jaw in relation to age, height, weight, and BMI ($p > 0.05$) (Table 24) and in relation to gender and ethnicity ($p > 0.05$) (Table 25).

TABLE 24: Comparison of the categorized measurements from Δ 90° to the lower posterior maxillary wall on the right side with age, height, weight, and BMI

Features	Δ 90° to the lower posterior maxillary wall						Value-p
	< 2			≥ 2			
	Avera ge	D.P.	Median	Avera ge	D.P.	Median	
Age (years)	67,0	19,8	67,5	61,1	16,1	63,0	0,2121
Height (meters)	1,7	0,1	1,7	1,7	0,1	1,7	0,4981
Weight (kg)	67,0	11,2	67,5	67,3	8,9	70,0	0,9341
BMI	22,6	3,0	23,2	22,4	2,9	22,8	0,8391

S.D.: standard deviation; 1: Student's t-test.

TABLE 25: Comparison of the categorized measurements Δ 90° to the lower posterior maxillary wall on the right side with gender and ethnicity

Features	Δ 90° to the lower back wall jaw				Value-p	OR	95% CI
	< 2		≥ 2				
	n	%	n	%			
Genre							
Male	15	*45,5*	18	*54,5*	0,2741	0,5	0,2 a 1,6
Female	17	*63,0*	10	*37,0*		1,0	
Ethnicity							
White	26	*55,3*	21	*44,7*	0,7851	1,4	0,4 a 5,9
Brown	6	*46,2*	7	*53,8*		1,0	

1: Fisher's test.

5.3.3.3. Left side - quantitative

No associations of the Δ 90° to the lower posterior maxillary wall measurement were observed with age, height, weight, and BMI ($p > 0.05$) (Table 26) and with gender and ethnicity ($p > 0.05$) (Table 27).

TABLE 26: Correlation between the measurement of Δ 90° to the lower posterior wall of the left jaw with age, height, weight, and BMI.

Features	r	Value-p
Age (years)	0,113	0,3891
Height (meters)	0,126	0,3381
Weight (kg)	0,132	0,3131
BMI	0,078	0,5511

1: Pearson's correlation coefficient.

TABLE 27: Comparison of the Δ 90° to the lower posterior maxillary wall on the left side with gender and ethnicity

Feature	n	Average	D.P.	Min.	1Q	Median	3Q	Max.	Value-p
Genre									
Male	33	1,6	0,4	1,0	1,5	1,5	2,0	2,5	0,9161
Female	27	1,6	0,5	0,5	1,5	1,5	2,0	2,5	
Ethnicity									
White	47	1,7	0,4	1,0	1,5	1,5	2,0	2,5	0,0831
Brown	13	1,5	0,6	0,5	1,0	1,5	2,0	2,5	

n: number of observations, S.D.: standard deviation, 1Q: 1st quartile, 3Q: 3rd quartile, 1: Student's t-test.

5.3.3.4. Left side - categorical

There was no association between the categorized measurements from Δ 90° to the posterior inferior wall of the left maxilla in relation to age, height, weight, and BMI ($p > 0.05$) (Table 28) and in relation to gender and ethnicity ($p > 0.05$) (Table 29).

TABLE 28: Comparison of the categorized measurements of the Δ 90° to and the lower posterior wall of the left jaw with age, height, weight, and BMI

Feature	Δ 90° to the lower posterior maxillary wall						Value-p
	< 2			≥ 2			
	Average	D.P.	Median	Average	D.P.	Median	
Age (years)	63,7	17,8	68,0	64,9	19,2	64,0	0,8081
Height (meters)	1,7	0,1	1,7	1,7	0,1	1,7	0,3451
Weight (kg)	65,7	9,5	68,0	69,2	10,8	70,0	0,1911
BMI	22,2	2,7	22,1	22,9	3,1	24,1	0,3711

S.D.: standard deviation; 1: Student's t-test.

TABLE 29: Comparison of the categorized measurements from Δ 90° to the lower posterior maxillary wall on the left side with gender and ethnicity

Features	Δ 90° to the lower posterior maxillary wall				Value-p	OR	95% CI
	< 2		≥ 2				
	n	%	n	%			
Genre							
Male	19	57,6	14	42,4	0,8952	0,9	0,3 a 3,0
Female	16	59,3	11	40,7		1,0	
Ethnicity							
White	26	55,3	21	44,7	0,5602	0,6	0,1 a 2,4
Brown	9	69,2	4	30,8		1,0	

1: Fisher's test.

6. DISCUSSION

The research for this work was developed after observing for approximately 10 years, during nasal endoscopic operations at the Hospital das Clinicas, UFMG, a constancy in the anatomical measurements discussed in the text, generally greater than 2cm. The measurements from the 90 degree angle to the posterior maxillary wall were the same regardless of gender, ethnicity, age, weight, or height, unlike other measurements that varied with such characteristics. A study is being developed at UFMG, performing the measurements in imaging exams (CT scans of the paranasal sinuses), observing the regularity of these exams.

Based on the observations in the operative practice, it was decided to perform the measurements on cadavers to confirm or exclude the observations, since no definitions regarding anatomical measurements were found in the medical literature. The proof of the regularity of these measurements allows a safe and constant anatomical reference with greater security in the approach to paranasal sinuses, especially taking into account the great anatomical variation of this region.In the measurements from Δ 90º to the posterior inferior and middle maxillary wall, values below 1.5cm were found as outlines. Such measurements are not accurate enough to be performed during the operation due to their anatomical position in relation to the Δ 90º, and are not feasible to be performed during the operations. Thus, we chose to use the measurement of 1.5 cm in relation to the upper point of the posterior maxillary wall at Δ 90° because it is more feasible and has no outlines.Table 3 shows the summary of comparisons with the respective statistical significance between the three measurements evaluated and the characteristics of interest stratified by side, with all p values > 0.05.

TABLE 3: Summary of the comparisons between the three measures evaluated and the characteristics of interest

Response Variables	**Side**	**Characteristics of interest (p value)**					
		Age	**Height**	**Weigh t**	**BMI**	**Genre**	**Ethnici ty**
Δ 90° to upper posterior maxillary wall (categorical or quantitative)	Law	0,814	0,681	0,217	0,081	0,482	0,987
	Left	0,762	0,225	0,976	0,415	1,00	0,304
Δ 90° to posterior medial maxillary wall (categorical or quantitative)	Law	0,268	0,643	0,746	0,916	0,585	0,802
	Left	0,480	0,342	0,194	0,347	0,517	0,501
Δ 90° to lower posterior maxillary wall (categorical or quantitative)	Law	0,068	0,295	0,967	0,502	0,317	0,800
	Left	0,389	0,338	0,313	0,551	0,916	0,083

No association was observed between BMI, ethnicity, gender, age, height, and weight of the cadavers in relation to the analyzed measurements. There were no associations between the measurement of Δ 90° to the lower, middle, and upper points of the posterior maxillary wall (categorical or quantitative) and any of the evaluated characteristics.

In the comparison between the right and left sides, there was a statistical association in the measurement of the midpoint of the posterior maxillary wall at Δ 90°, but this difference was only 0.2cm, with the right side being larger than the left side, which is not very significant when applied in surgical practice.

7. CONCLUSION

The analyses of the data presented in the text allow us to state that there is a fixed measurement between the posterior superior wall of the maxillary sinus and the 90 degree angle. The measurement found was always greater than 1.5cm, which may facilitate opening the sinuses safely during nasal endoscopic operations. The constant minimum distance of 1.5cm from the posterior maxillary wall to the base of the skull provides a correct and efficient opening of the posterior ethmoid sinuses and sphenoid sinuses. The measurements of the inferior and medial points in relation to the posterior maxillary wall should not be used in operative practice due to the difficulty of measurement because of their anatomical position.

No statistical association was observed in the difference between the Δ 90° to the posterior maxillary upper, middle, and lower walls, both categorically and quantitatively in any of the characteristics evaluated, i.e., the measurements are not influenced by age, weight, height, ethnicity, or gender.

The definition of the fixed measurement in the sinus anatomy in a region where there is a greater chance of iatrogenesis could allow surgeons greater safety and fewer complications in endoscopic nasal operations.

8. BIBLIOGRAPHIC REFERENCES

BUNZEN, D.L.; CAMPOS, A.; LEÃO, F.S.; MORAIS, A.; SPERANDIO, F.; NETO, S.C. Efficacy of endoscopic nasal surgery in the symptoms of chronic rhinosinusitis associated or not with polyposis. Revista Brasileira de Otorrinolaringologia. 72:242-246. 2006.

CASLER, J.D.; DOOLITTLE. A.M.; MAIR, E.A. Endoscopic surgery of the anterior skull base. Laryngoscope. 115(1):16-24. 2005.

HEMMERDINGER, S.A; JACOBS, J.B.; LEBOWITZ, R.A. Accuracy and Cost Analysis of Image-Guided Sinus Surgery. Otolaryngoly Clinics of North American. 38: 453–460. 2005.

JONES, T.M ; ALMAHDI, J.M.D.; BHALLA, R.K. ; LEWIS-JONES, H; SWIFT, A.C. The radiological anatomy of the anterior skull base. Clinical Otolaryngology. 27: 101–105. 2002.

KANTARCI, M.; KARASEN, R.M; ALPER, F.; ONBAS, O.; OKUR, A.; KARAMAN, A. Remarkable anatomic variations in paranasal sinus region and their clinical importance. European Journal of Radiology. 50: 296–302. 2004.

LUONG, A.; MARPLE, B.F. Sinus Surgery Indications and Techniques. Clinical Reviews in Allergy and Immunology. 30: 217–222. 2006.

LUBBE, D.; SEMPLE, P.; FAGAN, J. Advances in endoscopic sinonasal and anterior skull base surgery. South African Medical Journal. 98(8):623-5. 2008.

MUSY, P.Y.; KOUNTAKIS, S.E. Anatomic Findings in Patients Undergoing Revision Endoscopic Sinus Surgery. American Journal of Otolaryngology. 25(6): 418-422. 2004.

SCUTARIU, M.D.; BÂLDEA, V. Neighbouring relations of the posterior ethmoid studied by axial computed tomography. Morphologie. 94:51-57. 2010.

STAMM, A.C.; PIGNATARI, S.; SEBUSIANI, B.B.; GALATI, M.C.; MITSUDA, S.; HAETINGINGER, R.G. Endoscopic Computer-Guided Nasosinusal and Skull Base Surgery. Revista Brasileira de Otorrinolaringologia. 4:(68). 2002.

STAMM, A.C. Micro-endoscopic sinus surgery - basic concepts. Revista Brasileira de Otorrinolaringologia. 3: (68). 2002.

TAN, B.K.; LANE, A.P. Endoscopic Sins Surgery in the Management of Nasal Obstruction. Clinical Anatomy. 42:227-240. 2009.

TAN, H.K.K. Sphenoid sinus: An Anatomic and Endoscopic Study in Asian Cadavers. Clinical Anatomy. 20:745-750. 2007.

TAN, B.K.; CHANDRA, R.K. Postoperative Prevention and Treatment of Complications After Sinus Surgery. Otolaryngology Clinics of North America. 43: 769– 779. 2010.

TRIOLA, Mario F. Introdução à estatística. 9. ed. Rio de Janeiro: LTC, 2005

ANNEX 1: Identification Sheet

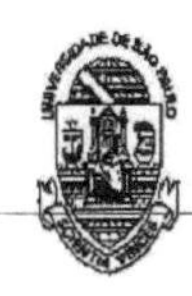

UNIVERSIDADE DE SÃO PAULO
SERVIÇO DE VERIFICAÇÃO DE ÓBITOS DA CAPITAL

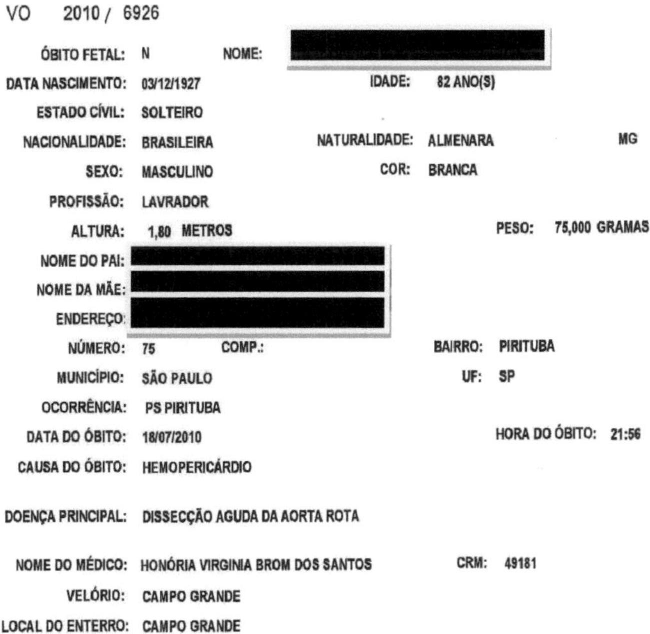

REGISTRO DE ÓBITO

VO 2010 / 6926

ÓBITO FETAL: N NOME: [redacted]

DATA NASCIMENTO: 03/12/1927 IDADE: 82 ANO(S)

ESTADO CÍVIL: SOLTEIRO

NACIONALIDADE: BRASILEIRA NATURALIDADE: ALMENARA MG

SEXO: MASCULINO COR: BRANCA

PROFISSÃO: LAVRADOR

ALTURA: 1,80 METROS PESO: 75,000 GRAMAS

NOME DO PAI:

NOME DA MÃE:

ENDEREÇO:

NÚMERO: 75 COMP.: BAIRRO: PIRITUBA

MUNICÍPIO: SÃO PAULO UF: SP

OCORRÊNCIA: PS PIRITUBA

DATA DO ÓBITO: 18/07/2010 HORA DO ÓBITO: 21:56

CAUSA DO ÓBITO: HEMOPERICÁRDIO

DOENÇA PRINCIPAL: DISSECÇÃO AGUDA DA AORTA ROTA

NOME DO MÉDICO: HONÓRIA VIRGINIA BROM DOS SANTOS CRM: 49181

VELÓRIO: CAMPO GRANDE

LOCAL DO ENTERRO: CAMPO GRANDE

S.V.O.C. - São Paulo, 22 de Julho de 2010

ANNEX 2: COEP approval

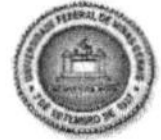

UNIVERSIDADE FEDERAL DE MINAS GERAIS
COMITÊ DE ÉTICA EM PESQUISA - COEP

Parecer nº. ETIC 0591.0.203.000-08

Interessado(a): Prof. Roberto Eustáquio Santos Guimarães
Departamento de Oftalmologia e Otorrinolaringologia
Faculdade de Medicina - UFMG

DECISÃO

O Comitê de Ética em Pesquisa da UFMG – COEP aprovou, no dia 24 de maio de 2010, após atendidas as solicitações de diligência, o projeto de pesquisa intitulado **"Estudo anatômico em cadáveres de pontos de referência endoscópio nasal ao acesso cirúrgico a base anterior do crânio"** bem como o Termo de Consentimento Livre e Esclarecido.

O relatório final ou parcial deverá ser encaminhado ao COEP um ano após o início do projeto.

Profa. Maria Teresa Marques Amaral
Coordenadora do COEP-UFMG

Av. Pres. Antonio Carlos, 6627 – Unidade Administrativa II - 2º andar – Sala 2005 – Cep:31270-901 – BH-MG
Telefax: (031) 3409-4592 - e-mail: coep@prpq.ufmg.br

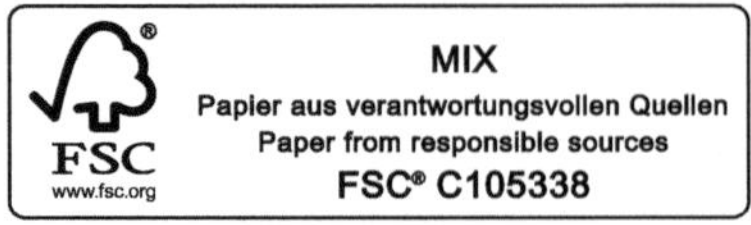

Printed by Books on Demand GmbH, Norderstedt / Germany